Herbs Th~~~~~

Hair-Loss &

Premature

Graying

Time-Tested Herbal Remedies

No Side-effects

by

Prayank

Contents

15. Liquorice ..

16. Mandukaparni for..

17. Neem for..

18. Vibhitaki for..

Some Important Guidelines

Introduction

Loss of hair from the head can mean baldness, a part of the wider topic of "hair thinning". Compulsive pulling of hair (trichotillomania) can also produce hair loss. Hairstyling routines such as tight ponytails or braids may induce hair loss. Both hair relaxer solutions, and hot hair irons can also induce hair loss.

Changes in hair color typically occur naturally as people age, eventually turning the hair gray and then white. This is called achromotrichia. Achromotrichia normally begins in the early to mid-twenties in men and late twenties in women. If it happens earlier, it is a sign of premature graying of hair.

In the book, you will find brief details of herbs that can be used to cure hair-loss and premature graying. It also gives you an option to choose the herb that is easily available in your locality.

Herb names may be different in different places, hence you should rely on botanical names to find how it is known in a particular place/location.

Though there are people who treat ailments inexpensively with herbal remedies, most consider it as the last minute miracle worker once all other avenues of treatments have been exhausted.

Such an approach discounts the sophisticated and elaborately documented information dealing with specific medicinal applications of herbs for specific complaints. The methods of herbal remedies are designed for optimum beneficial use and tested innumerable times in actual practice.

While every effort has been made to verify the authenticity of information contained in this book, it is not intended as a substitute for medicinal consultation with a physician. The publisher and the author are in no way liable for the use of information contained in the book.

1. <u>Almond</u>

(Pranus amygdalus)

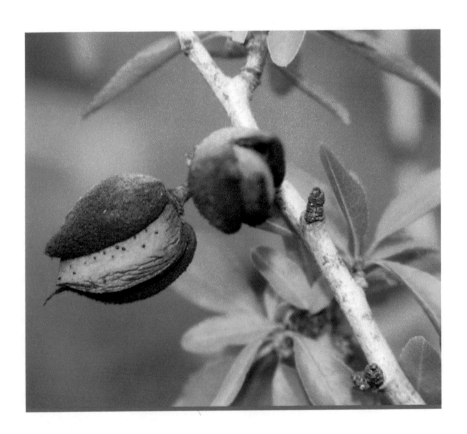

General

Almond contains twenty percent protein – a percentage one finds hardly anywhere else in the plant kingdom. Moreover, the quality of protein is such that it is easily digested. It is considered to be an ideal supplement to milk.

Profile

Botanical Name : Pranus dulcis, Pranus amygdalus, Pranus communis, Amygdalus communis

Family :

Appearance : A tree growing to the height of around 9 meters.

Medicinal Parts : Kernel, oil, shell

Distribution : The almond is native to the Mediterranean region of the Middle East, eastward as far as the Indus. It was spread by humans in ancient times along the shores of the Mediterranean into northern Africa and southern Europe and more recently transported to other parts of the world, notably California, United States.

Preparation and Dose

Apply a little almond oil on scalp frequently and massage.

2. <u>Aloe</u>

(Aloe vera)

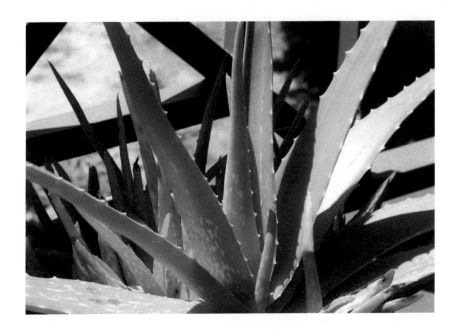

General

Aloe is a species of succulent plant that bears thorny lance-like leaves but is a favorite herb in beauty products. The fresh juice from leaves is yellowish in colour but acquires a brownish black colour on drying. The pulp is quite bitter to taste, and emits a somewhat offensive smell. It contains the active principle aloins.

Profile

Botanical Name : Aloe vera

Other Species : Aloe barbadenesis

Family : Liliaceae

Appearance : The fibrous root produces a rosette of succulent, lance-like leaves, whitish green on both sides with spines on the margins. Flowers - orange or yellow to purplish, in racemes. Fruit - a triangular capsule, ellipsoid-oblong.

Medicinal Parts : The gel-like pulp obtained on peeling the leaves and its dried form (powder); leaves.

Distribution : Widely cultivated throughout the world.

Prescription and Dose

Boil a mixture of equal quantities of leaf juice and gingelly oil (oil from sesame seeds) till all moisture has evaporated. Apply on the head and massage for a few minutes before retiring.

3. <u>Amla</u>

<u>*(Phyllanthus emblica)*</u>

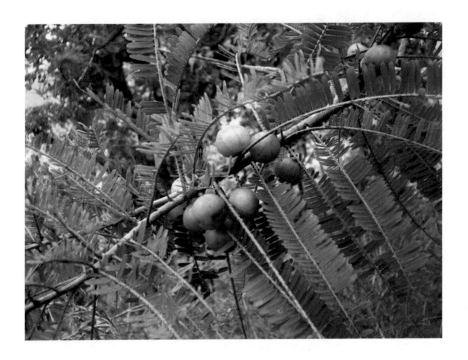

General

It is said that one can survive by consuming the fruit juice of amla only. It is the richest source of vitamin C, providing 3000mg of vitamin C per 100g of dried amla, which is heat stable.

There are two varieties of amla : the wild one with small fruits, and the cultivated ones with bigger fruits. Both are known to possess medicinal value.

Profile

Botanical Name : Phyllanthus emblica

Other Species : Emblica officinalis

Family : Euphorbiaceae

Appearance : A medium tree with smooth greenish-gray exfoliating bark. Leaves – feathery. Fruits – globose pale green, 1-5 cm in diameter, fleshy, sour in taste, 6-lobed.

Medicinal Parts : Fruits, leaves, flowers, seeds, root and bark.

Distribution : Native to India. It is present throughout tropical and sub-tropical regions up to 1500 m.

Prescription and Dose

Crush fresh amla fruit along with a little water and express about 2 teacups juice. Add to this equal quantity of cow's milk and juice of trailing eclipta (marsh daisy). Add 8 teacups coconut water and 6 teacups sesame oil. Mix in 3 tsp each fine powder of following separately:

Liquorice, wild turmeric, nutmeg, mace, chebulic myrobalan, belleric myrobalan, dried ginger and black pepper.

Now mix all the ingredients together in a vessel and heat over low flame. When the mixture reduces in volume and looses all traces of moisture, leaving behind a thick oil, remove from the fire. Allow it to cool. Bottle it.

Use 2-3 tsp of this oil to apply on scalp. Massage with fingers for 10 minutes. Wash it off with warm water.

4. <u>Calamus</u>

(Acorus calamus)

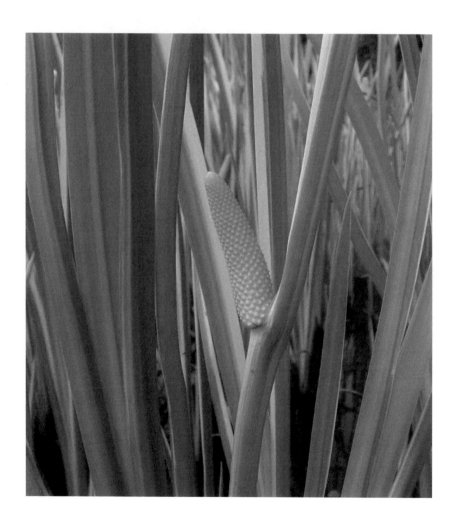

General

The scented leaves and more strongly scented rhizomes have traditionally been used medicinally and to make fragrances, and the dried and powdered rhizome has been used as a substitute for ginger, cinnamon and nutmeg. The dry rootstock yields a yellow coloured, aromatic, antiseptic volatile oil on steam-distillation.

Calamus oil is an acknowledged nerve-stimulant, helpful in mental concentration exercises. The oil is effective against a host of ailments such as gastritis and various skin diseases due to its antiseptic properties.

Profile

Botanical Name : Acorus calamus

Family : Araceae

Appearance : A marshy, fragrant herb. Leaves - simple, alternate, linear, glossy bright green. Flowers - fragrant, pale green on a stump. Fruit - a 3 celled fleshy capsule. Rootstock - pinkish brown, white and spongy inside.

Medicinal Parts : Rootstock (rhizome)

Distribution: Probably indigenous to India or Arabia, Acorus calamus is now found across Europe, southern Russia, northern Asia Minor, southern Siberia, China, Indonesia, Japan, Burma, Sri Lanka, Australia, as well as southern Canada and the northern United States.

Prescription and Dose

Mix 1 tsp powdered root in 2 tbsp cold coconut milk and make a paste. Apply on the affected parts and allow it to remain for 1/2 hour before rinsing it off.

5. <u>Carrot</u>

(Daucus carota)

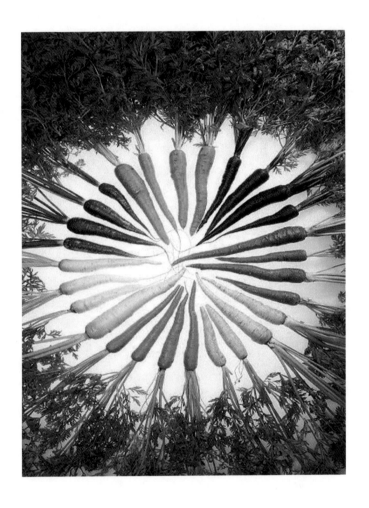

General

This common yet popular tuber can be eaten both raw and cooked. It contains good amounts of Vitamins - A, B and C besides starch, sugar, iron, calcium and phosphorous.

Profile

Botanical Name : Daucus carota

Other Species : Bee's nest, wild carrot

Family : Umbelliferae

Appearance : An annual or biennial herb. Stem - hairy and branched. Leaves - in fine divisions. Flowers - lacy white in clusters.

Medicinal Parts : Root(cultivated), leaves, seeds(wild)

Distribution : Generally available in most parts of world.

Prescription and Dose

Take a glassful of carrot, alfalfa and lettuce juices frequently.

6. <u>Chinese Hibiscus</u>

(Hibiscus rosa-sinensis)

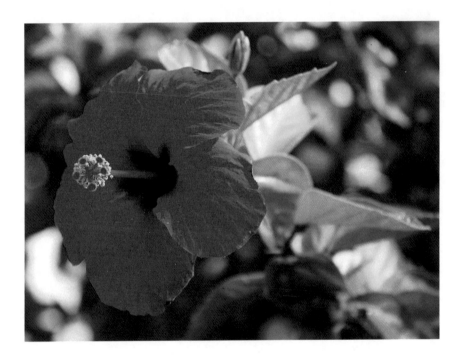

General

Chinese hibiscus is also known as Shoe-flower. It is cultivated as an ornamental plant in gardens.

It's flowers are astringent, hypoglycaemic, and considered to have an aphrodisiac quality. They are extensively used in treatments for alopaecia, burning sensation in body, diabetes, menstrual disorders, piles, fever, cough, menorrhagia and ulcer.

Profile

Botanical Name : Hibiscus rosa-sinensis

Other Species : Shoe-flower, Chinese rose

Family : Malvaceae

Appearance : Glabrous shrub. Leaves simple, alternate. Flowers of varying colours, often red. Petals five. Stamens numerous, united to form a staminal tube.

Medicinal Parts : Flowers, flower buds, petals, stamens, roots.

Distribution : It is native to East Asia, widely grown as an ornamental plant throughout the tropics and subtropics.

Prescription and Dose

Heat 10 flowers in 2 teacups coconut oil till charred. Filter and use as hair oil.

Note: Besides preventing hair loss, it also removes dullness of hair.

7. <u>Coconut</u>

(Cocos nucifera)

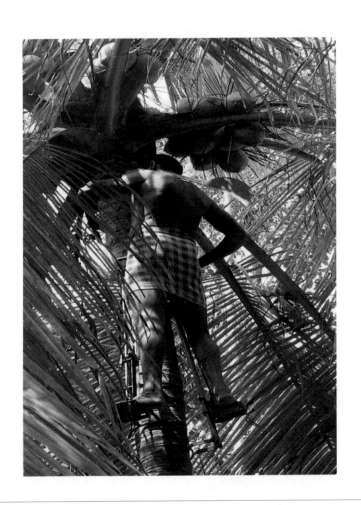

General

Coconut is considered a great preventive medicine. It is well known for its great versatility as seen in the many domestic, commercial, and industrial uses of its different parts.

The term coconut can refer to the entire coconut palm, the seed, or the fruit.

Profile

Botanical Name : Cocos nucifera

Family : Arecaceae

Appearance : A common tall palm growing up to 30 meters tall, with pinnate leaves 4–6 meters long, and pinnae 60–90 cm long; old leaves break away cleanly, leaving the trunk smooth.

Medicinal Parts : Leaf, fruit, oil.

Distribution : Found throughout the tropic and subtropic areas.

Ailments and Prescription

1. <u>Hair loss</u> - massage with coconut oil everyday.

2. <u>Thinning of hair</u> – grind ½ teacup each curry leaves, rinds of chebulic myrobalan and liquorice sticks into a fine paste. Boil this in 2 teacups coconut oil till solid mass chars. Filter and use as hair oil.

8. Curry Leaves

(Murraya koenigii)

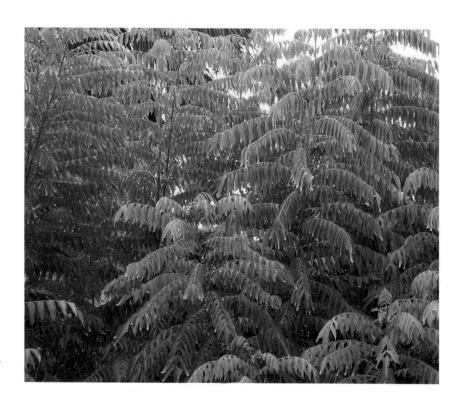

General

The curry leaves are germ-killers. The leaves in general, strengthen body, increase appetite, eliminate body heat and fever. The root-juice is consumed to relieve kidney pain.

Profile

Botanical Name : Murraya koenigii, Bergeria koenigii

Family : Rutaceae

Appearance : It is a small tree, growing 4–6 m tall. The leaves are pinnate, with 11-21 leaflets, each leaflet 2–4 cm long and 1–2 cm broad. They are highly aromatic. The flowers are small, white, and fragrant. The small red/black shiny berries are edible, but not their seeds.

Medicinal Parts : Bark, root-juice, leaves, fruit pulp.

Distribution: A tropical to sub-tropical tree is native to India.

Ailments and Prescription

1. <u>Falling hair, dandruff</u> - Mix equal quantities of dried curry leaves, lime peel, shikakai, fenugreek seeds and green gram. Grind them finely. Store and use as a substitute for soap or shampoo. It also helps in blackening the hair, and imparts shine to it.

2. <u>Premature graying of hair</u> – Take juice or chutney made of curry leaves every day, OR boil a few curry leaves in 1 tbsp coconut oil till charred. When cool, use as hair tonic to retain natural pigmentation.

9. <u>Fenugreek</u>

(Trigonella foenum-graecum)

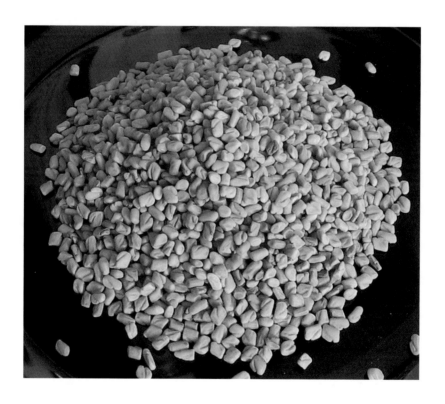

General

Fenugreek seeds are rich in iron and hence helpful in combating anaemia. It is also used to cure a number of common ailments – cough, fever, bronchitis, boils, ulcers..

Profile

Botanical Name : Trigonella foenum-graecum

Family : Leguminoseae

Appearance : Strong scented, erect, robust, annual herb with light green, pinnate, trifoliate leaves. Flowers – yellow. Pods – beaked. Seeds – brownish yellow with peculiar odour, oblong with deep groove across one corner.

Medicinal Parts : leaves, seeds

Distribution : Cultivated worldwide as a semi-arid crop.

Ailments and Prescription

1. Baldness, falling hair – Fenugreek seeds, ground in water and applied on the head. Allow to soak at least 40 minutes before washing. Every morning for a month.

2. Falling, dull, coarse hair – Fresh leaf paste applied over scalp before bath.

10. <u>Fig</u>

(Ficus carica)

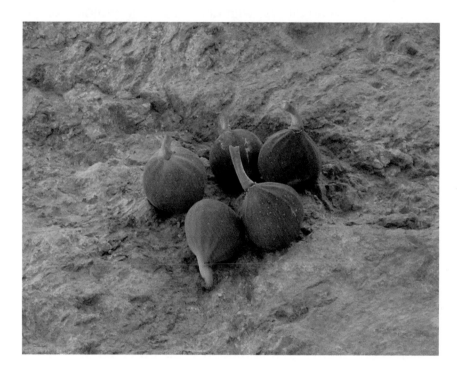

General

The fig tree which traces its origin to the Mediterranean region has enriched nutritional value. The dried fruits contain iron, copper and other minerals including trace elements like zinc, vitamin A and C, and a high concentration of invert sugar.

Profile

Botanical Name : Ficus carica

Family : Moraceae

Appearance : A small tree with alternate, long-petioled leaves. It bears its flowers inside a nearly closed receptacle. Fruits – pear shaped, fleshy. The stems and leaves contain an acrid milky juice.

Medicinal Parts : bark, leaves, leaf buds, roots, fruits (both fresh and dried), latex.

Distribution : Native to the Middle East and western Asia, it has been sought out and cultivated by man since ancient times, and is now widely grown throughout the temperate world.

Ailment and Prescription

Loss of hair – Dry out 2 teacups fig roots in the shade for 3 days. Crush them and immerse in 1 teacup coconut oil for 15 days. Strain and bottle. Massage on scalp at bedtime. Leave on overnight.

11. <u>Ginger</u>

<u>*(Zingiber officinale)*</u>

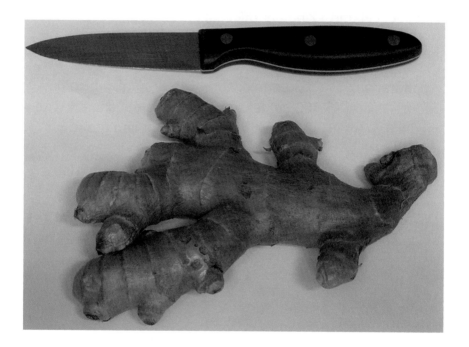

General

Ginger is referred as the universal medicine. Both fresh and dried ginger have almost identical medicinal qualities.

It lends its name to its genus and family (Zingiberaceae). Other notable members of this plant family are turmeric, cardamom, and galangal.

Profile

Botanical Name : Zingiber officinale

Family : Zingiberaceae

Appearance : Erect perennial herb with aromatic rhizome. Stem – erect, 15-150 cm tall, covered with leaf sheath. The sterile flowers are white with purple streaks and grow in spikes.

Medicinal Parts : Rootstock (rhizome)

Distribution : Ginger cultivation began in South Asia and has since spread to East Africa and the Caribbean.

Ailment and Prescription

<u>Premature graying</u> – Soak shredded ginger in honey. Eat a spoonful every morning.

12. <u>Haritaki</u>

(Terminalia chebula)

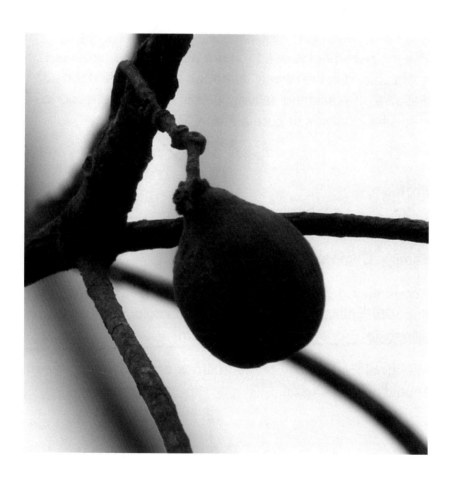

General

Haritaki, an indigenous tree of the Indian subcontinent has been in medicinal use for long. It is considered effective in many ailments. This tree yields smallish, ribbed and nut-like fruits which are picked when still green and then used for treatments.

The dry nut's peel is used to cure asthma. The bark/peel of the nut is placed in the cheek. Although the material does not dissolve, the resulting saliva, bitter in taste, is believed to have medicinal qualities to cure asthma.

Profile

Botanical Name : Terminalia chebula

Family : Combretaceae

Appearance : Tree with dark brown bark. Leaves - simple, opposite, shiny. Flowers - small cream coloured. Fruits - an ellipsoidal drupe, 5-angled, 4x2.5 cm.

Medicinal Parts : Rind of the fruit(raw or dried). Note - seeds should never be used.

Distribution: Native to southern Asia from India and Nepal east to southwestern China (Yunnan), and south to Sri Lanka, Malaysia and Vietnam. Found mainly in deciduous forests up to 1000m.

Ailments and Prescription

1. Graying of hair - Rinse hair with decoction of the fruit frequently.

2. Hair loss - Boil thoroughly a paste of 6 fruits in 1 cup coconut oil. Use this hair oil every day.

13. <u>Henna</u>

(Lawsonia inermis)

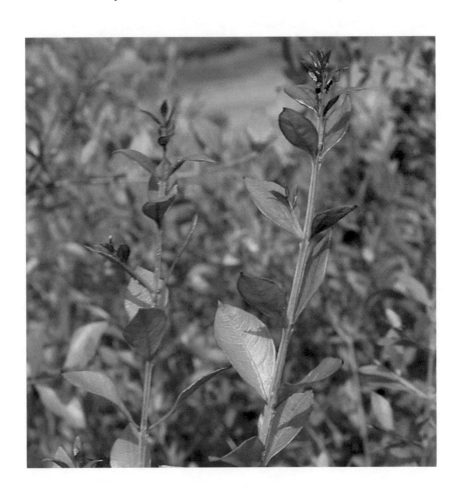

General

Henna is a flowering plant used since long to dye skin, hair, fingernails, leather and wool. The name is also used for dye preparations derived from the plant, and for the art of temporary tattooing based on those dyes.

Additionally, the name is misused for other skin and hair dyes, such as black henna or neutral henna, which are not derived from the plant.

The leaves, flowers and seeds of Henna plant have certain medicinal properties.

Profile

Botanical Name : Lawsonia inermis, Lawsonia alba

Family : Lythraceae

Appearance : A shrub or a small tree, with branches 4 angled usually ending in a sharp point. Leaves - green, also often with sharp points. Flowers - small, sweet-smelling, white or pinkish, in large bunches. Fruit - round, pea sized with many seeds.

Medicinal Parts : Bark, flowers, leaves, seeds.

Distribution: Native to Arabia and Persia. Now cultivated throughput India as hedge plant.

Prescription and Dose

Boil 2 cups gingelly or coconut oil. When oil is very hot, add a handful of henna leaves and allow it to splutter till it becomes red. Remove the burnt leaves from the oil. Use the same oil, add a fresh handful of leaves which will again splutter and turn red. Remove the burnt leaves and repeat the process for 2 or 3 handfuls more. Then allow the oil to cool and bottle it. Massage the head with this oil twice a day for 40 days.

(Note: The burnt leaves can be powdered and used as a medicine for treatment of burns, wounds etc.)

14. <u>Lime</u>

(Citrus aurantiifolia)

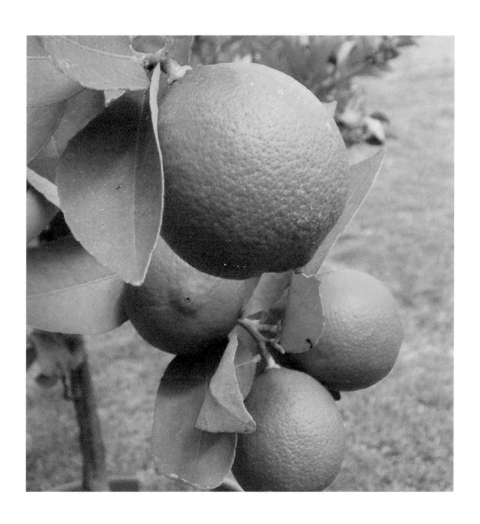

General

Lime is an easily available fruit, sour in taste and a rich source of vitamin C. They are grown all year round and are usually smaller and less sour than lemons.

Sour taste, in terms of herbalism, acts as a stimulant, promotes digestion, increases appetite and is a carminative (helps dispel flatus). It nourishes all tissues, except reproductive tissues.

Profile

Botanical Name : Citrus aurantiifolia, Limonia aurantiifolia

Family : Rutaceae

Appearance : A shrub or small tree. Fruit is typically round, green to yellow in colour, 3–6 cm in diameter, and containing sour and acidic pulp

Medicinal Parts : Fruits, Leaves, Roots

Distribution: Limes were first grown on a large scale in southern Iraq and Persia. Now, India tops the production list, followed by Mexico, Argentina, Brazil, and Spain.

Ailment and Prescription

Hair loss, premature graying - Mix dried rind of lime, with shikakai, curry leaves, seeds of fenugreek and green gram – all in equal quantities. Powder it and use for washing hair.

Or, grind 1 tbsp each pulp of amla with lime juice. Massage this into hair before going to bed. Wash it next morning with warm water.

15. <u>Liquorice</u>

(Glycyrrhiza glabra)

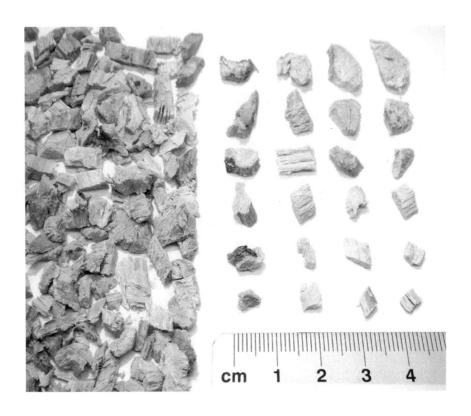

General

Liquorice or licorice is the root of Glycyrrhiza glabra from which a somewhat sweet flavor can be extracted. It has been known for thousands of years for its medicinal value. It is used to strengthen muscles and bone, curing wounds, bronchial troubles, skin diseases, ulcer and jaundice.

Profile

Botanical Name : Glycyrrhiza glabra

Family : Fabaceae

Appearance : Perennial plant found wild. The woody rootstock is wrinkled and brown on the outside, yellow inside and tastes sweet. The stem which is round on the lower part and angular higher up bears alternate odd-pinnate leaves. Leaflets are ovate and dark green in color. Flowers – yellow or purple or voilet. Pods – compressed.

Medicinal Parts : Rootstock(rhizome)

Distribution: Native to southern Europe and parts of Asia. Cultivated mostly in sub-Himalayan tracts.

Ailment and Prescription

Baldness, dandruff, hair loss – Grind 1 tbsp root pieces in 1 teacup milk with ¼ tsp saffron. Apply this paste on bald patches at bedtime continuously.

16. <u>Mandukaparni</u>

(Centella asiatica)

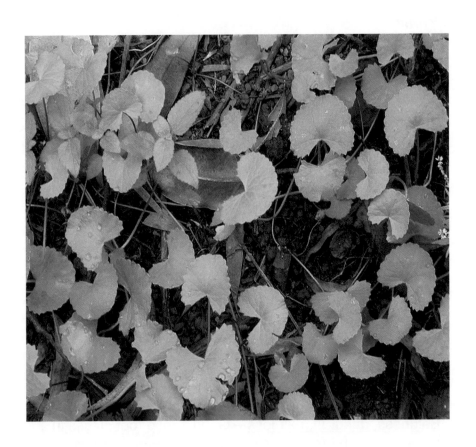

General

Mandukaparni in Sanskrit refers to shape and appearance of leaves of this plant, which resemble the webbed feet of a frog. The leaves also have a strong resemblance to human brain. The herb has been popular in the entire South East Asia besides China, Tibet, Japan and India.

Profile

Botanical Name : Centella asiatica

Other Species : Hydrocotyle asiatica

Family : Apiaceae

Appearance : A creeper bearing roots on nodes. Leaves - small, rounded/kidney shaped, with toothed margins. Flowers - pinkish red, minute, 3-6 in clusters. Fruits - small, 7-9 ridged.

Medicinal Parts : Whole plant - leaves, roots, seeds, stem

Distribution : Throughout India and SE Asia, in moist places, marshy banks of water bodies and irrigated fields.

Prescription and Dose

Mix equal quantities of centella leaf juice and coconut oil. Boil the mixture well. Cool and bottle. Use it as hair oil.

17. <u>Neem</u>

(Azadirachta indica)

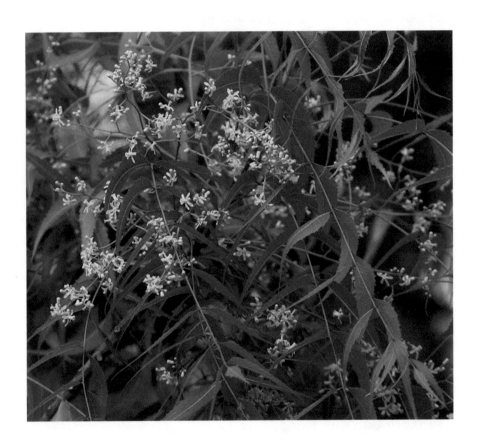

General

Neem trees are dedicated air-purifiers, constantly engaged in releasing pure oxygen into the air. Almost all parts of neem tree have some medicinal usefulness.

Profile

Botanical Name : Azadirachta indica, Melia azaderachta

Family : Meliaceae

Appearance : Deciduous tree up to 12 meters tall. Fissured dark gray bark. Pinnate leaves. Flowers small and white. Fruits green (yellow when ripe) with one seed.

Medicinal Parts : Flowers, leaves, bark, fruit, seed, oil, root.

Distribution: Native to India, Pakistan, and Bangladesh growing in tropical and semi-tropical regions.

Ailment and Prescription

<u>Dandruff, falling hair, lice, infection of scalp</u> – A handful of leaves boiled in 4 teacups water. After cooling and filtering, use this water to rinse hair.

18. <u>Vibhitaki</u>

(Terminalia bellirica)

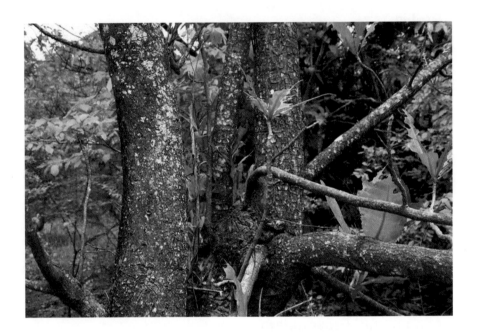

General

The fruits of vibhitaki exhibit hypotensive, purgative and choleretic activities. Its kernel is edible and is considered to have narcotic and aphrodisiac effects.

It is prescribed in a variety of diseases : anaemia, cough, fever, asthma, diarrhoea, dysentery, biliousness, diseases of eyes, nose and throat etc. It stimulates hair growth, cures leprosy, and purifies the blood.

Profile

Botanical Name : Terminalia bellirica

Family : Combretaceae

Appearance : A long avene tree with ash-grey bark, with patches of blue. Leaves - elliptic, crowded towards the ends of branches. Flowers - pale, greenish yellow with an offensive odour. Fruit - grey to light voilet when fresh, turning light brown later.

Medicinal Parts : Bark, fruits, leaves.

Distribution: Vibhitaki is a large deciduous tree common on plains and lower hills in Southeast Asia, where it is also grown as an avenue tree.

Ailment and Prescription

Premature graying of hair - Apply the oil extracted from seeds locally.

<u>Some Important Guidelines</u>

1. **Preparation**

When the herb is extremely bitter, sour, astringent or in powdered form, it can be mixed with honey, jaggery, sugar, candy etc.

2. **Dosage**

The quantity of dose can vary from one person to another based on individual age, physical build, and reaction of patient to a particular formulation.

The dosage prescribed in this book is meant for fully grown and mature patients. The dose should be increased/decreased for each patient keeping in mind individual patient's constitution.

3. **Effectiveness**

The contents of a herbal plant part varies widely due to factors such as climate, altitude, latitude, soil type, nutrition, temperature, relative humidity, time of plucking, packaging, storage etc. Hence the effectiveness of herb for treating an ailment may vary in different cases.

Patient needs to keep in mind this inherent weakness of herbal effectiveness, and be prepared to continue the treatment for a little longer time.

<u>Other Books That May Interest You</u>

Herbs That Cure:

Anaemia
Asthma
Bad Breath
Bleeding Piles
Constipation
Diabetes
Fatigue
Flatulence
Genito-Urinal disorders
Hair Loss
Insomnia
Joints Pain
Leucoderma
Obesity
Pimples
Psoriasis
Rheumatism
Sexual Debility
Toothache
Venereal Diseases
Wrinkles

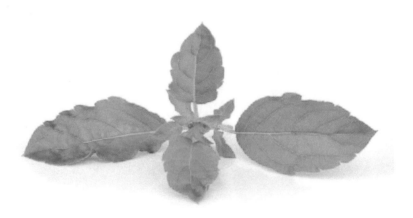

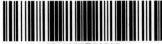

3613038R00030

Printed in Great Britain
by Amazon.co.uk, Ltd.,
Marston Gate.